THE CYCLE PATH

A STAGE MUSICAL

by Fiona Whelpton.

One million people commit suicide very year.
The World Health Organization

Published by:
Chipmunka publishing
PO Box 6872
Brentwood
Essex
CM13 1ZT
United Kingdom

http://www.chipmunkapublishing.com

THE CYCLE PATH.

A STAGE MUSICAL.

By

Fiona Whelpton

CAST OF CHARACTERS.

NARRATORS.

NARRATIOR 1.   A WHEELCHAIR USER.

NARRATOR 2.   A SIGNER

FIONA   (Aged 34) Her disability is caused by
anxiety.
She has periods of interrupted walking, and is
sometimes unable to use her arms.
Suffers from lack of confidence in herself.
Periodic episodes of speech deterioration.
Partially deaf.

DANIEL: (Aged 28) Artist. Alcoholic wildlife painter,
He crushed his leg in a motorbike accident. Hell's
angel. Bit of a Jekyll and Hyde personality.
Unpredictable behaviour, due to his drinking. Unable to

cope with his pain, both physical, and emotional. Can't stand up for very long, spends most of the time sitting. Either painting at an easel, or drinking heavily.

PETER (aged 19): MEDICAL STUDENT; Blonde from Cornwall. Kind, gentle, with a warm, Compassionate personality. Works extensively with Disabled people, in a special disabled people's residential Home. They absolutely adore him in the same way Fiona finds herself drawn to his magnetism. Loves children. Understands psychological pressures on Matthew.

MATTHEW   (aged 7-12): Aged 7 when play starts. Is 12 by the end of it. Is very hyperactive child with lots of excess energy and a bubbly personality.

FIONA'S MOTHER
MRS WHELPTON.   : Well-intentioned. Has always been there for Fiona. Basically a kind woman who has her best interests at heart. Over-protective because of the disabilities and mental illness.Constantly worried about her daughter, mainly due to her fear That she's venerable to the opposite sex. Patronizing and Domineering.

EXTRAS.   DISABLED PATIENTS.

CHILDREN IN HOLIDAY CLUB.

CHORUS OF

WHEELCHAIR DANCERS/ SIGNERS

ACT 11.

CHARACTERS

STAFF OF APPLE TREE COTTAGE.

PETER

MATRON

RESIDENTS OF APPLE TREE COTTAGE.

DIANE

MARGARET

THOMAS

ACT ONE   SCENES

SCENE 1 .   The Cycle Path

SCENE 2 Fiona's Kitchen

SCENE 3. Unity House Kitchen.

SCENE 4   Unity House Kitchen.

SCENE 5 Fiona's Kitchen..

SCENE 6.   The Living Room.

SCENE 7. Bedroom.

SCENE 8: The Cycle Path.

SCENE 9: Fiona's House.

ACT 11.   APPLE TREE COTTAGE. Home for disabled patients

SCENES

SCENE 1 . The Garden. Summer

Scene 2   The lounge.

SONGS

SONG 1   As we travel on life's journey.

SONG 2   We don't have to be different.

SONG 3   Why do I still love you?

SONG 4 The cooking Song

SONG 5 We don't have to be different (Reprise.)

ACKNOWLEDGMENTS

I would like to dedicate this musical to everyone who is disabled out there , also to everyone who has helped me to learn about live theatre .The cast of Theatrescape, Vanya ,Leila and Rosie from Indigo Brave theatre company who have taught me most of what I know about acting., Creative Routes for believing in me and giving me the confidence and opportunities to go out there and perform, Anna and Gaby from The Young Vic Theatre, for teaching me stage design skills .
I would like to thank Clive Millwater from Lost Artists Group for the cover photos, Jason Pegler and Andrew Latchford for their work on the editing, also Jamie Glaser for taking the time to read my work and supportive comments during a very busy recording

7

schedule. Finally I'd like to thank Penny Coulson and Theo Stickley from the NHS Arts development committee for the initial funding for this book, and everyone at Chipmunka publishing for believing in me enough to give me this opportunity.

The Cycle Path.

Stage, Musical.

STORYLINE SYNOPSIS

Fiona Whelpton, a disabled mother, with a young toddler, suffers from Conversion Syndrome Disorder. Her partner, Daniel, is an extremely talented wildlife artist, but is a compulsive alcoholic, which she is not aware of until she starts living with him.

Daniel's drinking becomes more serious, and he neglects her and her baby- to the point of becoming so resentful of them that he deliberately abuses her. He starts spending longer periods of time away from his family – preferring to rely on his mother, who sees herself as his saviour – but begins interfering in the relationship between him and his partner, because she is totally unable to let him go, because of his dependence on her. It twists and turns into a vicious spiral – ending up with his mother persuading him to move out.

He walks out on Fiona and the baby, leaving her to cope alone. She has to take out a court injunction, as he keeps trying to comeback, and she becomes more and more frightened for the safety of her baby and herself, even though he has made it clear that he is completely inadequate, and unable to take on any kind of adult responsibility. Fiona is left to make harsh choices between Daniel and her son, but she is aware of powerful emotions she is unable to stop.

As a result of a complicated delivery   Fiona begins to experience episodes of paralysis of the limbs, rendering her unable to walk for much of the time, or use her arms, at different periods of time, as well as deterioration of speech, and partial deafness,

Daniel's own problems with his feelings of inadequacy, are made worse by his serious drinking habits, which he uses to mask his pain, both emotional scars, and physical pain, with arthritis of his hip, and leg pain, making it difficult for him to sit, stand up, and manage stairs of any sort. He cannot sleep properly because of the pain, for long periods of time. Drinking is his escape route, but the subsequent hangovers make him cynical and nasty- tempered, mainly due to the problems he has sleeping properly because of being in pain at night time- especially if he doesn't drink late at night. This is the reason that he starts to drink more regularly, late at night, which makes Fiona's routine with a new baby impossible to deal with.

Daniel's mother tries to take over by making sure that she takes control of her son's spending habits, turning up on the doorstep every Tuesday, to make sure he doesn't spend all his money when he gets his benefits. She complains that Fiona isn't feeding him properly, even though meals are provided regularly, He just goes drinking, This becomes a sore point as his mother insists that he spends weekends at home with his parents, in order to prevent further drinking, because he can't cope with a screaming baby.

Fiona is scared of the choices that she faces – these are made harder by her physical pain, becoming more difficult, making every day life harder, especially now that her son is a toddler. He is likely to get into difficulty, because he is an avid climber. Her already acute anxiety made her much worse, and she starts experiencing blackouts on a fairly regular basis, as well as not being able to walk at different periods of time.

Her stress level is increasing as her baby turns into a lively toddler, and she relies on her Mum's help more and more.

She battles through her pain, but ends up collapsing while she tries to walk down the cycle path.

The play opens with her being found by a stranger.

The stranger is Peter, a 19-year-old medical student, who befriends Fiona and her son because he "wants to help."

Because of her vulnerability due to her acute loneliness she's suffered, Fiona finds herself aching for an outlet to express her emotions through him. She doesn't know how to respond to his gentle personality, which makes her feel as if she is a better person. In spite of talking sternly to herself, Fiona finds herself inevitably falling in love, but experiences real feelings of anxiety and guilt because of the massive age gap. She keeps her own age a secret.

She begs him to love her back, though she is unable to voice her needs, and shows him the way she really feels by reaching out to him – responding to his naturally affectionate nature, and warm, caring compassionate personality. Peter is used to relating to disabled people. His work shifts at the present time are involved in specializing in looking after disabled people with various disabilities, at a special care home. They really relate to him, and he helps their real personality develop by being willing to accept them the way they are. Fiona asks him to love her in spite of her disabilities; she hopes he will find true beauty as she feels he can see a beautiful person underneath. The feelings are unreciprocated. He rejects her. She is forced to face up to the truth about herself. This unblocks the fear. She grows through the experiences, learning to accept herself the way she is, doesn't need to pretend any more and finds freedom without a fairy tale Cinderella – type ending, but experiences transformation in a completely different way, which is

profound lasting, and life changing.

PROLOGUE:

NARRATOR 1. (ONSTAGE.)

SIGNER: (ONSTAGE)

OPENING SONG.

AS WE TRAVEL ON LIFE'S JOURNEY.

AS WE TRAVEL ON LIFE'S JOURNEY.

AS WE TRAVEL ON LIFE'S JOURNEY

IT TAKES US DOWN A PATH

OF RICH EXPERIENCES,

THAT MOULD US, AND MAKE US,

INTO THE PERSON THAT WE BECOME

AT THE END OF THE JOURNEY.

THE CYCLES MOVE FORWARD COMPLETING

LIFE'S CYCLE.

SO WE REACH OUR GOAL

AND HOLD ONTO THE JOURNEY OF

LIFE'S RICH PROMISES….

CHORUS:

RICH PROMISES, RICH PROMISES,

MAKE US WHO WE ARE

EVEN IF WE HAVE TO LOOK INWARDS

TO MAKE US INTO A STAR.

NARRATOR ! Is pushed by signer onto

(CENTRE STAGE.)

NARRATOR (1):

Having to cope with progressive disability, means
that one sees two sides of the coin, somehow, one has a
foot in the able- bodied, and the "disabled" world,

seeing everything from both perspectives, but from different angles, the same as everyone else, and yet not the same.

The "able-bodied – disabled " person whatever that means, (POINTING TO THE SIGNER) is automatically excluded, forced to be an outsider. (ANGRILY) People shut him out; ignore him, pretending that he doesn't exist. They see their own reflection in the mirror, and wonder what life might be like for them if they were in his place. (POINTING AT THE AUDIENCE) it might just be them, too. The "disabled person watches their reactions from his wheelchair.

(SIGNER MOVES TOWARDS WHEELCHAIR. SIGNALLING TO THE AUDIENCE AND POINTING DRAMATICALLY TN THE DIRECTION OF THE WHEELCHAIR.)

SIGNER:: Somehow, the barriers MUST come down. These fears and prejudices, which are based on sheer ignorance, prevent their victims from being everything they have the potential to be, because of our fears.

SCENE 1 THE CYCLE PATH

NARRATOR CENTRESTAGE Reading a letter.

Theme SONG As lights come up, revealing a
pathway onstage covered with leaves.

AS WE TRAVEL ON LIFE'S JOURNEY.

AS WE TRAVEL ON LIFE'S JOURNEY

IT TAKES US DOWN A PATH

OF RICH EXPRIENCES, THAT MOULD US,

AND MAKE US INTO THE PERSON THAT WE

BECOME

THE END OF THE JOURNEY.

THE CYCLES MOVE FORWARD

COMPLETING LIFE'SCYCLE.

SO WE REACH OUR GOAL

AND HOLD ONTO THE JOURNEY OF

LIFE'S RICH PROMISES.

SPOTLIGHT ON NARRATOR.

NARRATOR (1) Dear Peter,

I have missed you so much since you went away, and have not been able to stop thinking about you every single day. Matthew also misses you a lot, and keeps asking when you are coming back I don't know what to tell him, because I sense that you will not return. I know that I have really blown it, this time. I knew you were angry with me the last time that we saw you, because there was no connection there – nothing. After everything that we have been through together, you suddenly seemed so cold, and hard – and distant. I felt that I was trying to find someone who had once been there and existed no longer- I came away from that meeting and cried solidly for three hours. I knew that something was different and that it was never going to be the same again. I have never known you to be so cold towards me, but I knew that it must have been because of the baby – I would give everything to make things different, if I could turn the clocks back, I would. I wanted it to be perfect for us.

I love you.

Fiona.

NARRATOR 1: Dear Fiona,

Thank you for your letter- and many apologies to you for having taken so long to get in touch with you. As you can appreciate, I had my own reasons for doing this. I know that you are upset, but I don't think it's a good idea for us to be in continual contact now, as far as I am concerned, things are over between us. You are right to say that you feel that things can never be the same again. There is something that I should have told you, but I didn't want to hurt you. I am getting married to a girl I met at work. She's called Olivia. I hope that you can be happy for me.

I never wanted to cause you any pain, and hope that this will finally help you to put this in the past, and that you will be able to move on, as regards your thoughts of me.

Regards,

Peter.

LIGHTS GO ON, FOCUSED ON A BODY LYING SURROUNDED BY LEAVES AT THE BACK OF THE STAGE.

FOOT LIGHTS DIM ON NARRATOR AND FADE OUT.

ENTER PETER WITH HIS CYCLE STOPS, TRIES TO HELP FIONA.SHAKES BODY GENTLY, UNTIL SHE RESPONDS.

FIONA: (STARTLED)Who are you? What happened?

PETER: Thank goodness for that. My name is Peter, and I'm a junior doctor, actually, I'm just on my way to work. Can you get up?

FIONA: (TRIES TO SIT UP, PULLING HERSELF UP ON HER KNEES BUT IS UNABLE TO MOVE ANY FURTHER.)   I can't get up ………………….

PETER (OFFERING HER HIS ARM) Here- let me.

FIONA (GRABBING HIS ARM AND GINGERLY MANAGING TO STAND ON BOTH

LEGS, BUT IS SHAKING LIKE A LEAF) OUCH !

THAT hurt …………….

Peter: Do you remember what happened, then?

FIONA: Not really. Where am I? (LOOKS

AROUND) On the cycle path. I remember now – I was

going to Sainsbury's. , then I couldn't move my legs

properly – it's too steep , there's no way that I could

have managed to cope with getting down such a steep

hill in this amount of pain. Impossible. So I wanted a

quiet walk. The noise was making it worse, you see, it

always does.

PETER: It's just as well you didn't try to go any

further, then, isn't it? I doubt you'd have got far. Where

do you live? It can't be very far, can I help you get back

home?

FIONA: Would you? I'd be so grateful.

PETER: My pleasure. Here's my number. Call me later on. I'll just have to be late this morning

(LIGHTS FADE LEAVING STAGE IN DARKNESS.)

          *   *   *   *

SCENE 11. FIONA'S KITCHEN. (EVENING.)

(FIONA is trying to make tea, finding it really difficult to stand up to do things properly. DANIEL is sitting at his easel, painting on the other side of the room.

OFFSTAGE (TAPED BABY'S VOICE, CRYING)

DANIEL: For God's sake. (PUTTING DOWN HIS PAINTBRUSH,) Shut that fucking brat up. How can I concentrate with that entire racket that brat makes?

27

You are a hopeless mother – you can't even stop your own baby from screaming all the time. I'm surprised the neighbours don't send for the police,

FIONA: Do you think that you could do something to help? Those vegetables need chopping. Why don't you have a go at those, while I go in and see to Matthew, or you could always go and see if his nappy wants changing, and I'll finish making tea?

DANIEL: THAT'S woman's work!!!

FIONAA: (HANDING HIM THE SAUCEPAN) If that's woman's work, THEN TRY SOME OF THIS!!!!

DANIEL: (THROWING SAUCEPAN ON TO THE FLOOR, SPILLING WATER AND VEGETABLES EVERYWHERE) I'm not standing up chopping veg,

I'm NOT your servant,

FIONA: That's not fair- you're always treating me as if I'm yours. I don't even know why I bother cooking for you half the time as it is, because all you are interested in is fucking off to the pub for your next boozing session. I've had it up to here, inside this place on my own all day long, with nothing but a screaming baby for company, and you never talk to me any more, all you do is paint occasionally when you aren't drunk.

DANIEL: Bloody hell. Shut up, woman. Stop nagging me. Nag , nag , nag nag, you sound just like my bloody mother,. Well, you're right about one thing, forget the meal – I hate your boring dinners any way- my mum is a much better cook than you. At least she cooks proper food – you can't even boil an egg properly. I'm off. Don't bother waiting up for me.

FIONA: I'd given up waiting up for you long ago, but you and your wretched music wake both Matthew and me up. You might as well not even bother coming to sleep in the same room any more, get a camp bed, and move into the lounge. I'm not interested in sleeping with a hopeless drunk. Go on- why don't you get lost.

DANIEL: That's fine with me – just fine. I'm going to be away all weekend – I'm staying at Mum's

(SLAMS DOOR LOUDLY, LEAVING FIONA SITTING AT THE TABLE SOBBING, BABY SCREAMS LOUDLY OFFSTAGE.)

FIONA:(MOPPING HERSELF UP, TRYING TO TALK TO HERSELF CALMLY AND RATIONALLY.)

I would never have started a relationship with him in the first place, if I'd realised what he was really like. Everything just happened so fast – we felt really attracted to each other, and wanted to get married 24 hours after we met. Of course I knew that he is drank –

he was always one for going into the pub with his mates – he never gives me a second thought. What about me, then? Every time I try to help Daniel by doing nice things for him, like cooking, he throws everything back in my face. I love him so much. I can't bear it. I want to take his leg pain away from him, but there's no way that I can even do that. Anyhow, even if I did, then he'd just end up going back to his mother. I'm just ending up being a substitute mother, as far as he is concerned she makes sure that we can't have any kind of a normal family life. "Come for Sunday lunch" she tells him. But do they ever ask me over with him? Never. Not once.

I forgot to take my pain relief this morning. No wonder I'm so depressed. Sometimes I just end up with feeling like taking the whole lot and being done with it – no more pain, ever again. Well I'll just have to leave the mess on the floor. I can't bend over to pick anything

up. (BABY CARRIES ON SCREAMING) Forget the

cooking. I need to put him to bed.

EXITS.

THE KITCHEN THE FOLLOWING MORNING

.FIONA: Why can't I find my tablets? Daniel didn't come back until really late, as normal. I never saw him, but he woke me up playing his music full-blast.

(TELEPHONE RINGS SHE GOES TO ANSWER IT) Mum –

MRS WHELPTON: Are we going shopping today?

FIONA: Yes.

Mrs. Whelpton: Make sure you and Matthew are ready early, and I'll be over to fetch him.

FIONA: Thanks Mum. (PUTS PHONE DOWN BUT SHE THEN BEGINS TO STRUGGLE WITH HER WALKING.)

FIONA: I don't think I'll be able to go out today, I'd better try though. Maybe if I walk through the pain, I'll be able to carry on moving …… but right now, I don't know that I'll even be able to manage the stairs. If only I could find my painkillers. There's absolutely no sign of Daniel. Well if next try to get ready.

EXITS.

THEME SONG

 AS WE TRAVEL ON LIFE'S JOURNEY

AS WE TRAVEL ON LIFE'S JOURNEY

IT TAKES US DOWN A PATH

OF RICH EXPERIENCES, THAT MOULD US

AND MAKE US INTO THE PERSON THAT WE

BECOME

AT THE END OF THE JOURNEY.

THE CYCLES MOVE FORWARD

COMPLETING

LIFE'S CYCLE.

SO WE REACH OUR GOAL AND HOLD ONTO

THE JOURNEY OF LIFE'S RICH PROMISES.

*   *   *   *   *

FIONA'S KITCHEN..(FIONA COMES BACK

WITH MATTHEW, REALLY STRUGGLING AS

SHE TRIES TO GET HIS COAT ON,)

FIONA: Come on, Matthew, Granny will be here

in a minute.

MATTHEW (YELLING) I don't want to go out.

FIONA: You'll enjoy seeing Grin. Come on. She'll

be here in a minute.

MATTHEW; NO!!! (STAMPS FEET.)

FIONA; Matthew – I really don't want to have to

smack you – put your coat on.

MATTHEW: No. I WON'T. (STARTS

SCREAMING)

(KNOCKING ON THE WALL)

FIONA: That's the neighbour. Now see what you've done. You're nothing but a spoiled brat.

(LOUD KNOCK ON THE DOOR) That's Granny. (GOES TO OPEN THE DOOR. MRS WHELPTON STANDING OUTSIDE.)

MRS WHELPTON: Aren't you ready yet? I gave you plenty of warning. You could at least be ready on time.

FIONA: I haven't been able to get Matthew to do a single thing he's been told this morning. I can't walk properly this morning, either. Just take him. I've had enough.

MRS WHELPTON: What about the shopping?

FIONA: I don't think I can walk.

MRS WHELPTON: There are wheelchairs in there. We'll just have to use one of theirs. Get your walking sticks, and we'll be off.

ALL EXIT.

(CHORUS OF WHEELCHAIR USERS AND SIGNERS ONSTAGE.

WHEELCHAIR USERS…..SOME CAN STAND UP , SOME SIT DOWN. THOSE STANDING UP USING WALKING STICKS LIKE A FRED ASTAIRE STYLE CANE.

TAP DANCE.)

SONG: WE DON'T HAVE TO BE DIFFERENT.

DO WE HAVE TO BE DIFFERENT,

DIFFERENT FROM THE NORM?

DO WE HAVE TO BE DIFFERENT

TO BE ABLE TO WEATHER THE STORM?

WHY DO WE HAVE TO BE DIFFERENT,

BEFORE THEY HEAR WHAT WE HAVE TO

SAY

WHAT'S WRONG WITH "DIFFERENT"?

WHAT'S "DIFFERENT", ANYWAY?

I DON'T NEED TO BE ASHAMED

BECAUSE MY WALKING GETS IN THE WAY.

MY LEGS AND ARMS DON'T WORK THE

SAME

THE SAME AS YOU, AND ME

BUT EVEN IF THEY DON'T WORK RIGHT,

IT DOESN'T MEAN THAT YOU

CAN'T BEAR THE SIGHT

OR STOPS US STANDING UP TO FIGHT.

WE ARE JUST THE SAME AS YOU AND ME,

BUT "DIFFERENT"

BUT YOU JUST NEED TO SEE

BEYOND THE DIFFERENCE IS REALITY,

DREAMING OF WHAT I WANT TO BE,

AND WHAT I HOPE YOU'LL BE ABLE TO

SEE.

FIONA'S FRONT DOOR. (MRS WHELPTON,

FIONA AND MATTHEW STANDING OUTSIDE

WITH SHOPPING BAGS ON THE FLOOR..)

FIONA: I'll get my keys. (FUMBLES AROUND,

DROPS THEM ON THE FLOOR, STRUGGLES TO

BEND DOWN TO PICK THEM UP.TRIES TO PUT

THEM IN THE LOCK, BUT CAN'T)   I can't

unlock the door. Daniel must have locked it with his

keys. (SHOUTING AND KNOCKING) Daniel, can

you hear me? (NO RESPONSE .)

We'll have to go to the phone box.

MRS WHELPTON: I'll go. I think it will be easier if you and Matthew wait here.

EXITS. RETURNS SHORTLY AFTERWARDS.

MRS WHELPTON: I spoke to Daniel's Dad. He did come back to the flat. Daniel's Dad's coming over, he says we'll have to go and spend the night at my place – we have no choice. ((PICKS UP SHOPPING) How will he be able to get in?

ALL EXIT.

NARRATOR(ONSTAGE) When Daniel's father eventually managed to get into the flat, with the help of the police, who had to break the door down, they found that he had taken an overdose of Fiona's medication, and was unconscious, so he had to go to the hospital for a stomach pump, and stay there for a few days.

He also told Fiona that he wasn't coping – that he might have to move out altogether, but they decided to give things another chance. There was always another chance, and another, and another and another…………

It took Fiona a very long time to realize that she wasn't doing herself or her family any favours by giving him so many chances, sometimes it's like flogging a dead horse. But eventually Daniel made that choice for her. He disappeared with Matthew. She would never be able to trust him again, ever, and neither could her son, not only that, but it would make life so difficult for Matthew that he might find it impossible to ever trust adults again.

FIONA'S KITCHEN.

MATTHEW is sitting on the kitchen floor, eating his way through a whole packet of chocolate biscuits.

FIONA enters and finds her son with chocolate smeared all over his hands and face, looking extremely guilty.

FIONA: Matthew, what have you done?

MATTHEW

(LOOKING AT FIONA CHEEKILY .) It wasn't me Mum.

FIONA: Right. I'm at my wits end, or soon will be. I think we need to go out. You definitely need to be starting at nursery, once you can use the potty properly, you'll be able to, in fact the problem is that you need to be around the other children more already NOW, not in six months time. God, I feel so useless.

DANIEL: I'll take him out for you.

FIONA:: No you won't. He's MY baby – I have things to do. , You wait here. (EXIT). DANIEL

TAKES MATTHEW IN PUSHCHAIR. MATTHEW STATS TO SCREAM.)

FIONA, (RETURNING TO THE KITCHEN). I couldn't find them. Oh my God, they've gone. (PICKS UP THE PHONE)Mum, please come round, it's urgent.

(LATER THAT DAY, MOTHER ARRIVES ON THE DOORSTEP .FIONA IS GETTING MATTHEW READY:)

MATTHEW:Granny wouldn't ever hurt me, would she?

MRS WHELPTON: Darling, of course not. Granny and Mummy both love you.

MATTHEW : Daddy hurt me.

(FIONA AND HER MOTHER BOTH TURN PALE THERE IS A DEATHLY SILENCE .).

MRS WHELPTON: You mean to tell me that you left Matthew ALONE with THAT man? I sometimes wonder at you.

FIONA: I had no choice. He seemed fine.

MRS WHELPTON: That's just my point, though. That you never know whether he's fine or not , and then it's too late. . I am always so worried that he is going to hurt you or Matthew, or maybe both of you. You just don't know what he is capable of. How do you know what he might have done to Matthew, anything might have happened?

NARRATOR; How could she possibly live without knowing what happened? Maybe they'd never know. In any case, it was probably best for everyone, especially Matthew, not to know the real truth. Ignorance is bliss.

How can she forgive herself? She would have to live with the overwhelming guilt for the rest of her life. How can she still love a monster like Daniel? Because that's what he's become – a monster, of the violent sort, as well as the drinking, there's also the possibility that he could be a real child molester, Fiona mustn't allow him near her son, never EVER again.

MRS WHELPTON: I'm going to call the police.

FIONA: That's not your choice to make.

MRS WHELPTON: What choice do you have, Fiona? You are just going to have to choose between them. How can you ever be able to trust Daniel again, after this?

Matthew is totally dependent on both of you. He comes first. He has to.

(THE PHONE RINGS LOUDLY MAKING FIONA JUMP.)

FIONA: (Talking to someone on the other end of the phone) Where's Daniel? ~ I haven't seen him for a couple of days, and have been worried sick, oh; He's there now. Daniel, is that you?

DANIEL: Fiona, there's something I need to talk to you about, it's Matthew, I've hurt him. It's because I can't cope with stress of any sort , or any sort of responsibility any more. I've already been to the police and let them know, it's up to you if you want to press charges.

FIONA (SHAKING) Charges for WHAT?

LONG SILENCE.

DANIEL: It's OVER. I'm leaving you.

(FIONASITS DOWN, SHAKING.) I feel sick. (PUTS HEAD BETWEEN HER KNEES) Mum, phone

46

the health visitor, I can't, can't, can't cope, cope, cope, cope....

NARRATOR: Daniel was taken by the police for further questioning, but remained silent throughout. They couldn't press charges because they failed to say:" Anything you say may be taken down in evidence." A court case was arranged and happened a year later. Fiona was granted a residency order, as they decided it was in Matthew's best interests to stay with her. They took out an injunction to stop Daniel coming within thirty yards of them. If he turned up at any playgroup, nursery, or school, he'd be arrested immediately.

SONG: WHY DO I STILL LOVE YOU?

WHY DO I STILL LOVE YOU,

EVEN WHEN YOU CAN'T BE TRUE?

AND LOVING YOU IS MAKING ME BLUE?

YOU ARE JUST NO LONGER YOU

AND I DON'T KNOW WHAT TO DO.

BECAUSE I JUST CAN'T STOP LOVING YOU

IT'S MAKING ME FEEL SO BLUE.

BUT I HAVE TO MOVE ON

TO SOMETHING NEW

BECAUSE MY JOY HAS GONE

AND ALL THAT'S LEFT FOR ME

 IS SINGING THIS SONG.

SPOTLIGHTS ONSTAGE PREVIOUS SCENE

FADING OUT.

NARRATORL

Dear Fiona,

I hope you are starting to recover from some of the blackouts, and that they have started to subside. Can you remember the first time I saw you? It had been on my way to work on the cycle path; I always choose that way, because it is so much quieter than walking up the bridge, and along the main road, where it is so noisy at that time in the morning. I love the cycle path in the autumn in particular, because there are so many different colours in the leaves, as they turn russet, gold, brown and orange. The pyranthia bushes along the cycle path look wonderful as I cycle past them on a crisp, frosty morning.

It was completely unexpected to find someone lying there. It is so unusual; especially to come across somebody unconscious as you had been, that day. The strangest thing about the situation was that the paralysis kept coming and going, and I felt so

49

sorry, because you were obviously in a great deal of pain. My job as a Doctor is to help people get better, or at least cope with pain But in your case, I felt completely useless. My first responsibility, if I couldn't do anything for you personally, was to get you appropriate medical help. At least your house wasn't very far away from where you fell. You are incredibly brave. It must be so frightening not to be able to feel anything underfoot.

My apologies for suggesting that you walk to the car, it was completely insensitive.

I hope that by now you are more comfortable, and that you have started to be able to move around a bit more, Do let me know, without any hesitation, if there is anything that I can do to help you. I will contact you soon.

Yours,

Peter.

SCENE 111 UNITY HOUSE KITCHEN..

FIONA: When I looked at Peter as he offered to carry me to the house, it seemed as if he were connecting to my personality. He has a way of looking at you really closely. I love the way that a warm smile lights up the whole of his face. It's funny with some people, even though you've only just met, they don't feel like strangers. That's how it was with Peter. I felt completely at ease with him, even though it had been starling to find him bending over me when I wasn't too sure what had happened to make me fall over unconscious.

I'd never had a blackout before, and couldn't remember anything, either. But I felt so secure, and warm and safe when he lifted me in his arms. Somehow it felt wrong to ask him into the house, bust as soon as he had gone up the cycle path, I deeply regretted not having asked him in.

Peter was so different from any other men that I knew, Charming, very polite, caring and handsome. Even though my vulnerability meant that I had no choice but to let him go, I was conscious of how desperately I wanted him to say.

He made sure I was safe, and then had to leave, making me feel lonelier that ever. I felt such a sense of inevitability throughout the whole of that morning, and now I found myself longing to hear from him again.

I feel much more content about everything than I normally do, after having to deal with one of my episodes of paralysis. Usually I find it really hard having to be alone, and the burden of too much physical pain makes it even harder to bear.

Whenever I become physically disabled, I find myself fighting a whole mixture of different emotions, because there are so many walls between anyone who is able-bodied and me. There is an immediate sense of isolation. Most people don't know how to approach me when I become ill. They stare at me, coldly, and walk straight past, not wanting to get involved. When I get home, I always seem to turn the blame in on myself. If I were like other people, I would be able to make contact straight away, but there are so many problems caused by the simple fact that I can't stand up to have a normal conversation for any length of time. I put up barriers of shyness .It prevents people who try to talk to me from becoming too close. I do this because I am frightened of being found out,

NARRATOR :: Sometimes the disability can almost be an advantage. To the outsider, it is immediately a disadvantage, but for the person behind the disability it can be used to its full advantage. One can "pretend" to be helpless. One can hide behind the "mask." There are very few people with whom disabled people feel comfortable enough to show their real self. If they want to look beyond; the mask that's up to them. When illness strikes, people don't even usually bother to come and help, they are too embarrassed.

FIONA: That's why this morning had been so unusual, and why I haven't been able to stop thinking about the young man. Usually, it takes a long time before I can start moving around again properly, but today was different. I felt cheerful, almost hopeful about life. I am even starting to feel more positive. What was even stranger was that I didn't tell anybody, not even my mother, about what had happened that day.

We have since seen Peter several times, he knows just how to handle Matthew, and always calms me down.

SCENE 1V: UNITY HOUSE KITCHEN.

(FIONA AND MATTHEW ARRIVE AT THE
FRONT DOOR OF UNITY HOUSE.THEY GO
STRAIGHT THROUGH TO THE KITCHEN
MATTHW SCREAMING.)

FIONA::I almost feel guilty about feeling like this,
because I just don't know how old Peter might be. My
guess he's at least twenty. In any case, I must be a great
deal older than he is. So I am going to say anything to
him about it, and I certainly won't tell him that I am
really attracted to him. He'd run a mile.

I don't think Peter is the sort of person
who'd actually mind a great deal, actually- age is really
irrelevant, and anyway .Not if you like each other, and I
get the feeling that he does really like us.

Why is it that when he goes away I end up feeling lonelier than ever? Why do I like him? He's charming, very polite, caring, and as well as handsome. The first time I met him there was a sense of inevitability about everything, as though something was meant to be. But I shouldn't be longing to hear from someone I hardly know again, like this, should I? I hate myself for being disabled. It makes me angry.

SPOTLIGHT ON NARRATOR AND SIGNER ONSTAGE.

NARRATOR: We fight a whole mixture of emotions about being disabled. It's easy to hate ourselves. It's easier to hate ourselves for being different, rather than love ourselves and accept ourselves the way we are – That's much more challenging.

The problem is the immediate sense of isolation. Most people shy away from approaching anyone disabled, they stare at you coldly, and walk straight past, desperately trying to avoid you. Then the damage is done when we blame ourselves for something that isn't really our fault. There are so many problems caused by just the simple fact that it is often impossible to stand up and talk to anyone for any length of time without too much physical pain. The problem is the barriers of shyness so many put up to prevent people from becoming too close. We push them away out of fear – fear of being found out. But sometimes the disability can almost be an advantage – to the outsider though, it is immediately a disadvantage, but for the person behind the disability it can be turned to its full advantage. One can hide behind the mask. There are very few people with whom we feel comfortable enough to show our real self

UNITY HOUSE KITCHEN.

CHORUS OF CHILDREN ONSTAGE WITH COOKING UTENSILS ETC……

THE COOKING SONG.

BEAT, BEAT , BEAT , BEAT……….

MIX, MIX, MIX, MIX…

STIRRING THE SPOON, STIRRING THE SPOON,

BEAT THE MIXTURE , BEAT THE MIXTURE

DRUMMING AND HUMMING TO THIS TUNE.

MIX THE FLOUR, MIX THE DOUGHT

KNEAD WITH FISTS SO NICE AND SLOW

DON'T BEAT IT TOO ROUGH,

MAKING PUFF PASTRY

USING A MICROWAVE MAKES EVERYONE LAZY………..

CRUNCHY BISCUITS, SOFT SPONGES…

JAMMY DODGERS, ICED BUNS…

CHEESE SCONES, RAISIN SCONES

SCONES WITH JAM AND CREAM………

BUT MY FAVOURITE IS BAKING

HOME- MADE BREAD,

RISING HIGHER THAN I'VE EVER

SEEN………

BEAT , BEAT, BEAT , BEAT……..

MIXING, MIXING, MIXING, MIXING……..

MAKING IT SWEET……

ROLL OUT THE DOUGH,ROLL OUT THE

DOUGH……..

STRECHING IT AS WE SING THIS

SONG...........

NARRATOR OFFSTAGE (READING A

LETTER.)

Dear Fiona,

I hope you are starting to recover

from some of the black-outs, and that they have started

to subside. Can you remember the first time I saw you?

I remember it very well. It had been on my way to

work, on the cycle path . I always choose that way,

because it is so much quieter than walking up the

bridge and along the main road, even when it is so

noisy at that time in the morning. I love the cycle path

in the autumn in particular, there are so many different

colours in the leaves as they turn russet, gold, brown

and orange, The bushes look wonderful covered in red

berries as I cycle past them on a crisp, frosty morning. It was completely unexpected to find someone lying there. It is so unusual, especially to come across somebody unconscious, as you had been that day. The strangest thing about the situation was that the paralysis kept coming and going and I felt completely useless. My first responsibility, if I couldn't do anything for you personally , was to get you appropriate medical help. At least your house wasn't very far away from where you fell. You are incredibly brave. It must be so frightening not to feel anything underfoot.

My apologies for suggesting that you might be able to walk to the car. It was completely insensitive. I hope that by now you are more comfortable and that you have started being able to move around a bit more. Do let me know if there is anything I can do to help you and Matthew,

Yours Peter.

ENTER FIONA . (BREATHLESS AND ANXIOUS . PETER PICKS UP ON HER ANXIETY THEY STAND , STARING INTO EACH OTHERS EYES.)

PETER; What's wrong? Where's Matthew?

FIONA: I can't feel my legs, and he's run off. I'm scared. I can't move fast enough to go looking for him, or even keep up with him . I can't cope any more.(BURSTS INTO TEARS. PETER HUGS HER.)

PETER: Come inside, have a cup of tea while I go and look for him. CUP OF TEA.

PETER EXITS. SOMEONE MAKES FIONA A WHILE SHE SITS, REFLECTING.

FIONA: He's such a sweet man. His eyes are so radiant. They are such a radiant blue. Why do I feel so emotional? It's like a waterfall bubbling around inside me, what's it about? Someone being kind and gentle towards me. I can't handle it. I just don't know how.

Somehow I expect everyone to be horrid to me. My life's always been full of "if only's" What will be, will be.

PETER ARRIVES ONSTAGE WITH MATTHEW.

FIONA: Oh, thank goodness. Where on earth have you been?

MATTHEW: I went to play in the churchyard, Mum.

FIONA : But you know full well not to run off.

PETER: Leave it now. It's YOU I'm bothered about. You look shattered. Tell you what, why don't I come back home with both of you, and then Matthew and I can play football outside, and you can have a break for a while? You need to wind down,.

FIONA :I'm so grateful, You've been so kind to us, really. I don't know what I would have done if anything had happened. It would have been all my fault. I feel so responsible.

PETER: Everything is not always your fault. Come on, I'll take you home.

ALL EXIT

SCENE V FIONA'S KITCHEN.

(FIONA IS PREPARING LUNCH. LOUD KNOCK.

FIONA GOES TO ANSWER THE DOOR MRS WHELPTON IS OUTSIDE.)

MRS WHELPTON: Aren't you going to let me in? Where's Matthew?

FIONA: Outside.

(MRS WHELPTON PUSHES PAST, LOOKING OUTSIDE THE KITCHEN WINDOW.)

He's a very handsome fellow. He's very blonde. Looks German. Is he ?

FIONA: No. He comes from Cornwall. Actually, he's a medical student.

MRS WHELPTON: He looks so young, He's only a boy. Do you know how old he is?

FIONA: I don't know.

MRS WHELPTON: Then if you won't ask him, I'M going to .If he's going to spend any amount of time with MY grandson ,then things like that are important. Hasn't he got the most expressive eyes, though?(FIONA LOOKS EMBARRESSED) I have another question. How come somebody who is as attractive as he is, is still single at his age? I would have thought most people would have found him impossible to resist, not with looks like that.

FIONA: As far as I know, he has never had a girlfriend.

MRS WHELPTON: (GOING EXTREMELY PALE) what??? Do you think that there's any possibility that he might be gay?

FIONA: For goodness sakes, Mother. I never heard anything so outrageous in my entire life. Peter would absolutely NEVER be any of those things that you dare say about him. Get out , You are making me too stressed out.

MRS WHELPTON: All right, I will leave, but be very careful about the amount of time that you let him spend with Matthew, alone, until you know more about him than you do now, It takes a very long time before you know somebody properly. (WALKS OUT IN A HUFF, SLAMMING THE DOOR. ENTER PETER.)

Peter: What's wrong?

FIONA: It's nothing, really

PETER; It doesn't look like nothing.

(SITS NEXT TO HER LOOKING INTENTLY AT HER.)What did your mother say that upset you?

FIONA: My mother gets very possessive if anyone gets involved with me and Matthew. She finds it very difficult to trust any men, and even questions their sexuality. Just because she has had bad experiences with relationships, she thinks everyone else will be the same. But it has been so hard on our own, without any help. Sometimes it just gets impossible when he is so lively, and I can't move fast enough to be able to make sure that he doesn't come to any harm . I have been so much happier now I am no longer alone.

PETER :I'm here. And I am not going anywhere. You've had a really bad time. You know I will always be here for you . You know what the situation's like, and what my job involves .I know you have Matthew, and I realise how hard it is for both of you. I know it must be very hard for you both. A boy needs a man around, and if there is anything that I can do to help you and Matthew, then I will.

(FIONA STARTS TO FEEL MORE AWKWARD)

FIONA: I think Matthew and I need to be on our own for a while.

PETER: Don't worry, everything will be fine. I'm on nights over the next few days, but I will see you soon. If you want me to spend time with Matthew, just let me know, and I will be here for both of you. I have to go.

FIONA(REFLECTING) I know these feelings that I am starting to have, are completely inappropriate He doesn't even know how old I am. I know I really should tell him. It's best to be honest, isn't it; after all, what's the point of trying to have a relationship with someone you can't even trust? But what happens if he finds out that I haven't told him anything, and if I do tell him everything about me and Matthew, then he just won't want to know me anymore anyway, so I might as well avoid trouble, and not say anything. This age thing – somehow it's going to be very important, and yet in another way, it really shouldn't matter –to either of us. Just because it matters to my mother. I don't know how long I can keep my feelings hidden. It must be obvious. Peter is so understanding. He'd be more upset by the fact that I feel unable to trust anyone, and that includes him, even though he's been so kind to us. As an individual he seems more humane than anybody else that I have ever met. I don't have enough confidence in myself, and it wouldn't take much to completely destroy what little self-confidence I do have. Mum's right. I don't know him well enough . I wish we had more time on our own. Why are relationships so complicated? It's barely worth getting involved at all. Most men I get involved with stay around for a while, and then they just disappear. Although it would really help Matthew to have a man with Peter's personality around .Mum's said:" If you don't tell him, I will" So how can I live with that constant fear? I already have a knot in my stomach and feel sick most of the time, it's affecting my health. Thank goodness its bedtime and I can have some time to myself.

EXIT.

FIONA: ONSTAGE . (REFLECTING.)

Peter accepted the invitation to dinner. I wonder whether I should have a candlelit dinner and really spoil him, on the other hand, perhaps not, it might be too obvious. When I feel well, cooking is one of life's pleasures. It' nice to be giving something back to somebody else, but how can I make him feel good without it being too obvious? I think if you live alone, home cooking is always welcome. Peter is different. He can cook very well, which makes it harder to decide. He probably thinks he should be cooking me a meal.

I am really looking forward to this, almost TOO much. I have never felt so excited about anything before seeing him, I feel like a small child opening presents On Christmas Day. The happiness becomes overwhelming. I can't wait to see him again.

SCENE V1 THE LIVING ROOM.

(PETER AND FIONA SITTING VERY
CLOSELY TOGETHER ON THE SOFA.)

FIONA: It was really difficult to know what you
might enjoy the most. Most men don't know how to
cook, but I know it's one of your main hobbies, quite
an unusual one,

PETER: What makes you think it is so unusual,
then?

FIONA:(PAUSING,CAUTIOUSLY) Daniel never
took the slightest interest in eating together as a family,
let alone helping. He said it was "woman's work."

PETER; Maybe that's true in some families, But
Mum always made a point of including all of us in what
she was doing. Take bread-making, for example. How
do you think I learned to do it? It was because she let
me watch her make it while she did it, and then she let

me try for myself. I know Matthew hasn't had the chance of any positive male input like that, and that is one of the main reasons I wanted to help, not to mention the fact that my younger brother is his age, Young children are such hard work. Mum was always on her own with us.

FIONA (SHOCKED) Really? I didn't know.

PETER: Well, Dad was always working away, really. He was in the army, you see, based in India. He was always away, travelling. They might have well have lived separate lives. She might have well have been in your situation.

FIONA You are the first man I have ever met who feels men should have an equal amount of responsibility when it comes to domestic duties. Daniel would never lift a finger, and just disappeared off to the pub, even when he could see that I was struggling to

give him a nice meal, and sort out a screaming baby at
the same time.

(SILENCE. PETER LOOKS AT FIONA
INTENTLY.) You've had a bad time, haven't you?

(FIONA: LOOKS AWAY,)

NARRATOR: Fiona was scared of giving too
much of herself away to him. The question of the age
difference was fast becoming part of her wanting to
protect her privacy. It had reached the stage of
becoming the "big" secret .She is eventually reminded
of her mother's threats which have succeeded in putting
the fear of God into her., and already attempted to bring
up the subject naturally, but had become so fearful of
the outcome once Peter had discovered the truth about
why she and Matthew were on their own, then she
started clamming up completely, feeling sick every
time the subject got mentioned. Once the conversation

took a turn for the word, the pain in her legs would become much worse. She felt as if there were a giant skeleton in the cupboard, the cupboard of her secret past, and that Peter had the key to unlock the secrets, Fiona desperately needed to be able to trust somebody for once in her life, and felt that she could trust Peter. But the pain that was there at the very thought of what he might end up thinking about them was totally unbearable, and the direction in which the conversation turned, made her cringe.

PETER; Tell me some more about Daniel, I forgot what you said he did.

FIONA: Daniel didn't do anything, He was a complete loser. He was a very talented artist. He used to paint wildlife before he had an accident.

PETER: What accident?

FIONA: Well, a few years ago, he became a Hell's Angel. He bought himself a motorbike. Anyway, to cut a long story short, a car went into the back of him, he came off, and damaged his right knee, and now he is in permanent pain. That was the start of all his problems. Because of his pain, he started drinking to much.

PETER: Isn't it funny how different people's temperaments are?

FIONA: Yes, I had noticed.

PETER: Take you and me, for example. You are so much more tense than me, and emotional, but maybe that is what I like about you. I am too predictable, and I like surprises. Every time I see you, there is something new to discover.

(THE FRONT DOOR BANGS LOUDLY.)

FIONA (RISING) That'll be Mum, with Matthew.

(GETS UP TO ANSWER THE DOOR, MRS
WHELPTON AND MATTHEW OUTSIDE,
SCREAMING.)

FIONA: What's the matter?

MRS WHELPTON: Your son. He's what the
matter is.

I never thought I'd hear myself say this, Fiona, but
I just can't cope any more. He is completely beyond
me.

FIONA: It's not Matthew's fault.

MRS WHELPTON: Well, you try having him
around all the time, screaming and screaming and
screaming. I must have tried everything to get him to
stop, and nothing would. These Mothers have
absolutely no idea of the effects that they have when
they leave their child with someone else.

FIONA: It isn't as if you are a complete stranger.

MRS WHELPTON: That doesn't mean that it's the right thing to do, and a child of Matthew's age has no other way of letting the adults know they don't want to be left. The poor little mite was screaming until he was blue in the face.

FIONA: It isn't as though I'm out at work all day. I just wanted to talk to Peter on our own, for once.

MRS WHELPTON: Peter is much more important to you than your own son It is obvious that he means everything to you. You are always ready to drop everything else. I have already done my but, I've been though everything with you while you were growing up, and I never expected to go through it all over again.

FIONA: For goodness sake, calm down, otherwise Peter will hear you.

MRS WHELPTON: I don't care if he does.

(PETER COMES INTO THE HALL)

PETER: What's wrong?

FIONA Nothing.

MRS WHELPTON: NOTHING?? Do you know that I have to give up all my time to help Fiona out?

PETER: I don't think that Fiona has actually got a great deal of choice in the matter. I was only thinking that it was a good thing that Matthew has got a granny who could help out, otherwise there us no knowing what might happen to him, what with Fiona struggling with her pain every single day. I'm sure most of us haven't got a clue. It's about time we were more sympathetic. Instead of being ready to condemn disabled people all the time, they have enough to cope with, just being disabled, without any of the extra pressure. Fiona needs to know that she can count on you.

MRS WHELPTON: How DARE you ! Of course my daughter knows she can count on me. I am the one who has been left holding the baby, and putting the pieces back together from all her messes. Remember that I don't have anyone to support ME when things are difficult;. I've had to learn to stand alone in the last 16 years. I have already gone through bringing up my own family, and wasn't expecting to start all over again at the beginning .Fiona; you were not in a position to have a baby. How could you have been so irresponsible, as to have bought a child into the world when you should never have had him? He ought never to have been born.

FIONA: I can't take any more of your criticism. I am sorry that I haven't been the perfect daughter , but at least I have tried to keep going, and have always tried my best for Matthew.

PETER: Shouldn't that be our main priority here? Surely all this shouting is not good for him, or either of you, come to that. Come on , I'll make a cup of tea and you take some deep breathes and calm down.

MRS WHELPTON: I don't need to be told to "calm down" by somebody who has just come out of short trousers.

(FIONA MAKING DRINKS IN THE KITCHEN, REFLECTING, RETURNS TO SEE PETER AND HER MOTHER WITH ARMS AROUND EACH OTHER, EMBRACING.   SHE DROPS THE TRAY, AND RUNS OFFSTAGE, CRYING..)

SPOTLIGHT ON NARRATOR: Fiona couldn't believe her eyes. She kept telling herself to stop being so stupid and irrational. She had been feeling so guilty for being half Peter's age, but this was completely ridiculous. Her own mother falling into the same trap.

She couldn't cope any more. Feelings of complete rage and jealousy were raging around inside her. She wanted to lock herself away from all human contact and remain alone, forever. She should never have trusted anyone, after all , she couldn't even trust her own mother any more. But the biggest mistake she made trusted herself. She felt incapable of making a mature judgment, and couldn't judge anybody's character. She obviously didn't have a clue, she'd never be able to trust anybody again. Human beings are complex creatures when it comes to matters of the heart. Emotions run so high, that it becomes difficult to separate them from logic. Women are much more emotional than the majority of men seem to be, They seem much more capable of staying in control and maintaining the good old British stiff upper lip . As for showing someone you really care, that's just too risky. One must never show the other person how you really feel. You might get hurt, but I know there is a great deal of truth in saying that you must never trust anyone TOO much, even the people closest to you. They have the capacity to hurt you too much, much more than you'd ever imagine. Fiona felt she was a completely naïve idiot, who could be taken for a ride by every opportunist.

SCENE V11 BEDROOM

NARRATOR: That night, Fiona started experiencing new physical symptoms.

She lost the ability to speak completely. Unable to move any part of her mouth, because of the weakness in her face, and she was absolutely petrified. She knew she'd been wound up. Even her mother didn't know how to deal with the situation. Things were bad enough. At least she'd been able to use her time for reflection.

FIONA: Surely Mum couldn't really fancy him? How can she do this to me? She's so concerned about me; she's hardly likely to be interested in Peter in the slightest. He's so sympathetic to everyone; he has a real gift of empathy. He probably was only giving her a shoulder to cry on. He wouldn't dream of encouraging anything, not Peter.

But I can't forget how distressed it's made me feel.
I have no claims on his attention. We've never
discussed our friendship going any further .It doesn't
matter any more, because I certainly won't be haring
from him again, after this. If he hasn't been put off by
what he's seen, then he definitely been put off by all the
things she said. He probably thinks we are a completely
dysfunctional family, if he goes now, and never comes
back, it jolly well serves you right. She accuses me of
making messes all the time. It seems to be the only
thing I'm good at. All this is totally ridiculous. She's
done so much to help me. She's always been there for
me. She'd always been there for me, she wouldn't ever
dream of hurting me on purpose. I'm the problem. It's
my entire fault. I miss her. I need her more than ever.
Oh God, the postman's bought a letter. It must be from
him. (OPENS LETTER)

Dear Fiona,

I don't know what I've done that's

upset you so much. I was upset for both of you. It

seems that your mother really cares about you, and only

has your best interests at heart, you know, All she

wants is the best for you and Matthew. I did enjoy

yesterday. It was so nice to have some time together.

Have to be at work this morning. Do phone me on the

mobile. I'm really worried about your loss of speech.

There was nothing going on as far as I was concerned. I

was comforting her, she was in such a state. If I don't

hear from you, I will come round and talk to you over

the next few days. Try not to worry too much, and I

hope you are talking again, soon.

Yours Peter.

Fiona: we really need to talk. This is getting way

out of my control. The relationship's gone way beyond

making impressions. We need to walk somewhere quiet, down the cycle path, sit somewhere by the canal, maybe have a picnic. I'll call Peter and ask him.

SCENE V111 THE CYCLE PATH.

FIONA: (FIONA GETS OUT PICNIC RUG AND BASKET. PETER AND FIONA SITTING TOGETHER IN SILENCE, FIONA WATCHING HIM , INTENTLY)

PETER: Fiona, may I ask you something, I know it's personal, but why do you think your speech came back when I contacted you?

(NO REPLY .PETER DRAWS FIONA TO HIM SHE PUTS HER HAND ON HIS SHOULDER. THEY KISS. FIONA PUSHES HIM AWAY.)

FIONA: Peter, we mustn't. I can't.

PETER: Why? I have grown to understand you. I feel protective towards you. What's wrong with showing you that I care?

FIONA: It isn't that. I can't do this Peter. You don't understand.

PETER: Understand what? If it's about being disabled that's the worst reason there is. If I found someone attractive it doesn't make the slightest difference.

FIONA: It's nothing to do with that. But my disability is completely unfair on you. I just can't have a relationship and expect you to accept the limitations that I have to live with every day, Peter; I couldn't do that to you. I just love you to much. You deserve something so much better.

(BURSTS INTO FLOODS OF TEARS.)

PETER: Do you really think that matters, now? Of course it doesn't. I have always been there for you, haven't I? Doesn't that say something?

FIONA; Yes, I suppose……………

PETER L Well what's wrong with showing somebody that you care, then?

FIONA: Because the physical side is dangerous. One day I'll tell you. Let's just stay friends.

PETER: I know that's not what you really want, Fiona. (HE MOVES TOWARDS HER, LIGHTS START FADING OUT)

FIONA: You don't love me, you don't love me………………

(STAGE IN DARKNESS.)

SCENE V1111 FIONA'S HOUSE.

(FIONA IS LYING AT THE BOTTOM OF THE STAIRS, UNABLE TO MOVE.)

DIONA: Matthew, help me.

MATTHEW: Mummy, what's the matter?

FIONA: I can't get up.

MATTHEW: Shall I get help?

FIONA: Get the ambulance, NOW.

MATTHEW (ON THE PHONE) it's my Mum She can't move. Ambulance please

THE SPOTLIGHT GOES ONTO THE NARRATOR ONSTAGE.

NARRATOR: The paramedics arrived and helped her get to the hospital where she had more tests. This time she was in shock because they told her she was pregnant. She tried to contact Peter for weeks, but got no response. All she could do was wait.

FIONA'S KITCHEN. (KNOCK ON THE DOOR. FIONA GOES TO ANSWER IT TO FIND PETER STANDING OUTSIDE.)

PETER: Aren't you going to let me in?

FIONA: Did you get my messages?

PETER. Yes, But I've been away, working in Warwick. I'm here for a month, then I'm off to America for a year. Anyway, how are you, and how's Matthew?

FIONA: There's something I need to tell you. I've been really ill over the last few months, and they've found something.

PETER; What have they found?

FIONA: I'm pregnant.

PETER: How can you possibly be, I haven't heard from you for months.

FIONA: As far as I'm aware, it only takes the once what happened before you went away?

PETER: Oh, THAT! FIONA: what are we going to do, Peter?

PETER: I would have thought the best thing in your situation would be to have an abortion. You really have no other choice.

FIONA: I can't believe I am hearing you say this. You're a doctor. I wouldn't have thought you'd tell me to take a life.

PETER: I can't help you.

FIONA: Why not, you wanted it too?

PETER: Yes, Ok I admit it. But things have changed. I'm not going to be in Nottingham much longer.

FIONA: So where are you going, then?

PETER: I told you. To America, for at least a year. I have already signed a contract, and there isn't anything I can do now...

FIONA: There's something I have to tell you. We have to talk.

PETER: So what do you need to tell me, then?

FIONA: I love you, Peter.

PETER I Know, I think I always knew.

Fiona. Do you think marriage is a viable option?

FIONA: what, are you asking me to marry you?

PETER: No I don't love you. I can't ever marry you.

FIONA: there's something else, Peter. It's my age. Do you know how old I am?

PETER: I'd say about 35.

FIONA. Add on 10 years to that. (SHE IS NOW DOUBLING UP IN AGONY FALING ON THE FLOOR.PETER HELPS HER ONTO THE SOFA.)

PETER: So that's what I didn't understand.

FIONA: Yes, that you are half my age. But I still love you.

PETER.:You've GOT to forget me. You've just GOT to.

FIONA: How can I when I can't stop loving you, anyway what about the baby?

PETER: I told you before, have an abortion, I'm not going to be around, in fact, I had better go now and never come back.

(WALKS THROUGH THE DOOR SHUTTING IT QUIETLY BEHIND HIM LEAVING FIONA ALONE ONSTAGE, STUNNED.)

LIGHTS FADE LEAVING SPOTLIGHT ON
NARRATOR.

NARRATOR: That was the last time she ever saw
him. She had the abortion, but ever since she told him
everything, told him the truth, she has walked normally
with now pain. The paralysis has gone completely, and
she can now do things that she could only dream of
before.

ACT 11. APPLE-TREE COTTAGE. HOME FOR DISABLED PATIENTS.

SCENE 1:(THE GARDEN. SUMMER. THE PATIENTS ARE SITTING OUTSIDE HAVING AFTERNOON TEA. THE TABLE HAS A PRETTY TABLECLOTH AND PROPERLY SET WITH CHINA CROCKERY AND PLATES OF SANDWICHES.

ENTER MATRON. CARRYING A BIG FRUIT CAKE.)

MATRON: You're in luck this afternoon, Margaret, it's a Dundee cake.

(PUTTING THE CAKE DOWN ON THE TABLE) Did I tell you we're expecting late arrivals for tea?

MARGARET: That'll be something extra-special to look forward to, won't it?

MATRON: We're expecting them any time now, you can pour tea out, seeing that it's your turn to be mother, and I'll go and listen out for the door.

MARGARET (TURNING TO DIANE.) who do you think she might be bringing to see us today, then?

DIANE: Well, I don't know, do I.? How should I know? You know what it gets like in here; Matron always ends up treating us all like little kids. I do wish that she wouldn't talk down to us in such a patronising tone of voice, all the time.It really gets on my nerves, actually.

MARGARET: Stop moaning. Matron's very sweet, she really cares about us. We're not badly off in here, you know, it could be much worse. They try to do everything they can to make us happy, here.

DIANE: Well, if that's the case, I don't know what any of the other places must be like. I think everyone should be cared for by their own families, actually, and then the rest of us could have our peace and quiet and enjoy our old age in peace.

MARGARET: I wouldn't worry , you have a long time to go before you can be called "old" in any sense of the word, actually.You're young yet, but I know I'm no spring chicken .

DIANE: That'll be one up for this week's tribunal, minus one, for your prejudiced attitudes young lady.

MARGARET: I don't need to be called "A young lady" by somebody who is young enough to be my daughter.

DIANE: Age is relative, anyway. They all treat you as if you are two years old. That's another one for the tribunal.

(WHIPPING OUT A NOTEBOOK.) I'd better make a note of all this, now. Best make sure you don't waste the rest of your life being made to feel like some dumb idiot, just because all your physical faculties don't work the same way as everybody else's. It doesn't mean that our minds don't work properly, either. People are just so ready to become completely prejudiced against us. They never see further than their own narrow-mindneess, and making assumptions that are really harmful to us, without bothering to ask us how we feel about things.

MARGARET: I'm sure nobody really intends to talk to us as if we don't exost, or treat us like babies; it's just that they don't really know how to relate to us. Well. Maybe we can tell everyone how to relate to us. Hey need to see us and our issues differently. They need our help to shed light on things.

DIANE: How do you propose to get everyone listening to us, then? What about all those people out there? (POINTING TO THE AUDIENCE) Don't you realise how you make us feel intimidated. Maybe Peter will talk to them . They'll soon listen to what he's got to say about it all, far more than anyone else.

ENTER MATRON: Here are your visitors. Please make them feel welcome and Diane, remember not to get over huffy and offensive if anyone says something to you that you don't agree with.

(ENTER CHORUS OF WHEELCHAIR USERS AND ABLE-BODIED DANCERS WHO ARE CARERS, TOGETHER WITH MATRON AND PETER.)

PETER: How is everyone? Good to see you folk looking bright and cheerful today. We've bought some very good friends of ours to come and meet all of you.

DIANE: (GLOWERING AT HIM) How can you call them "friends "of ours, when we've never met them before in our lives? Even you patronise us. Do you fancy going up for the tribunal, next week?

PETER: Diane! You know how fond I am of everyone here, Can't you see that I only have your best interests at heart?

DIANE: Why is it that you youngsters think that you know everything? We've been around at least twice as long as you have, and yet you are always talking down to us like idiots.

Right. Haul him up before the tribunal, folks! We're not having this!! We don't have to put up with such rubbish!

PETER: Have a nice cup of tea, Diane, it will calm your nerves. There, there, there, you'll upset yourself. How about a nice piece of Dundee cake?

MARGARET: Give her that Dundee cake, for goodness sakes, then perhaps she'll stop moaning. Moan, moan, moan, moan, and moan. That's all she ever does around here. We get fed up of her. YOU get away from it, when you go home in the evenings. WE don't, or can't. You have to mind your P'S and Q'S around here, especially with this patient's tribunal. What happened to "please and thank you?" No wonder the children these days haven't any manners. They don't have any role models after all.

MARGARET: There's two of them up for the next tribunal .At least they sit up and take notice of how you feel .(TO THE AUDIENCE) what about you, then? Will you just continue to stay comfortable, and not change at all? Do you even want to?

MATRON: SILENCE! You leave them out of it. They've come to enjoy themselves.

DIANE: Yes. At our expense.

PETER: Shall I go and ask them what they think?

MATRON: All right, then. We need to get their opinion. Why don't you go right ahead and ask.?

PETER: We might as well, I suppose. After all, nothing is going to keep you lot quiet, an we're getting fed up of all the constant criticisms, when all we're trying to do is help all of you have better lives. Oh, well!!! What it is to be appreciated!!!!!!(SIGHS) I'll just go and fetch a microphone then. (EXITS OFFSTAGE. RETURNING WITH MICROPHONE) Right, then, am I expected to do this by myself, or is anybody game for coming down there with me? No, I thought so. I'll just get on with embarrassing all those poor folk out there, who have just come out for a nice night off. I wish I could get a night off, soon, I need a break to do something else that might stop me worrying about you lot all the time.

PETER WALKS DOWNSTAGE INTO THE AUDIENCE, HOLDING THE MIC. HE APPROACHES A VARIETY OF MEMBERS IN THE AUDIENCE AT RANDOM.

PETER: (TO AUDIENCE MEMBER) so then, what do we need to do to se these matters right for those guys up there? Do you think staff do their jobs well, or well enough? Are there things they might be able to do better, perhaps?

DIANE (ONSTAGE) Just listen to him, who does he think he is, Freud?

PETER: Diane, give us a break. We are already fully aware of YOUR opinion of all staff. Maybe you should sop roles for a little while, and see how you would cope with everything that we have to do. We want to get a broader picture on all of this.

(TO AUDIENCE MEMBER 1) Thank you, that's interesting. What do the rest of you all think? Do you think people become more disabled, depending on the way that others treat them? By the way, we are having a party tonight, and everyone is invited to come to see just what we get up to. You might learn some new things about disabled people that you have never had the chance to see before.

(TO AUDIENCE MEMBER 2) So – you think disabled people cause their own problems with communication skills, then? Don't you think it's because everyone is too busy these days to bother to communicate via body language, etc? That matters, you know. Maybe those guys feel awkward in the body that they have to express themselves in, and outsiders end up picking up on their awkwardness, making things even more uncomfortable than they already are. I think folk feel patronised because some of them are too proud to ask for help, actually, and then they feel awkward, which is then passed on to everyone else.

What can we do to make sure people feel as if they are a decent human being?

DIANE: STOP IT!!!!!

PETER: Stop what?

DIANE: Stop treating us all like two- year olds, why can't we go down there and talk to the audience, instead of having somebody talking FOR us, we have mouths of our own, don't we?

PETER: No-one could help noticing that about YOU , Diane, why don't you walk down here on your own, then?

DIANE:That's enough cheek from you, young man, You should know by now that I can't walk anywhere without being pushed. So who's going to want to push me down there?

MARGARET: The way you're acting now, I'm not surprised nobody wants to help.

DIANE: WHO asked YOU? I never asked to be helpless, having to spend all day and every day stuck in this thing, being ignored most of the time, and having to cope with being totally dependent on the goodwill of others, whether I want to be helped or not. What choice have I got?

MARGARET: You have a choice about the surly look on your face that's there all the time, and is a real put-off .Being rude certainly doesn't help anybody, even if they want to approach you to help, out of kindness,

DIANE: I have a choice, do I? Really, I don't think so.

MARGARET: Look at the way you are always so horrible to Peter, here. It's not ok, you know. He works far harder than anybody else I know, and he DOES listen to us.

DIANE: In that case, none of the others have the right to be horrible to us, either- we are always reminded of being worse off than anybody else, because people have an attitude problem the minute they see that we can't move around like they do – it's as if everyone who has a pair of arms and legs that work properly is automatically better than we are, and I am sick to death of being reminded of what I can't do. What about focussing on what I CAN do, instead? People don't think there is a person sitting in the wheelchair.

MARGARET:I wasn't aware that ayone was being horrible to us in here, actually. I think you are so upset by the way outsiders have treated you over the years, that you automatically expect everyone else to treat you the same way, even if they are responding totally differently to us. I think you almost invite rejection because you expect to be pitied. I know life doesn't seem to be very fair on those of us without all our faculties, but we can help others by being positive and cheerful instead of always moaning on and on and on ……Peter's right.

DIANE: At least he can walk out of here, when the going gets rough, we just have to put up with living with at least one person we can't stand.

MATRON: Now, now, children………I think it's a completely inappropriate place to be talking about things like this in front of complete strangers.

DIANE: At least he can walk out of here when the going gets rough.WE just have to put up with living with at least one person we can't stand.

: Here we go, first of all , they are everybody's friend, and now they suddenly become complete strangers. Does the woman think that we've gone completely off our trolley?

MARTON Let's treat our visitors as guests should be treated, come and have some our fruit cake and tea. You are most welcome to our party later, too.

DIANE: Haven't you forgotten something?

MARGARET: What, now?

DIANE: The tribunal, of course. Why don't we do it tonight, then our guests will have the chance to find out what it's really like in here, and we can all go mad and celebrate.

MARGARET: Well, we all went mad a long time ago. Ok then, if that's all right with you, matron?

MATRON: Let's do it after supper then, before getting ready for the party.

TAP DANCE WITH WALKING STICKS,

SCENE 11 THE LOUNGE PARTY.

SONG WE DON'T HAVE TO BE DIFFERENT.

DO WE HAVE TO BE DIFFERENT,

DIFFERENT FROM THE NORM?

DO WE HAVE TO BE DIFFERENT

TO BE ABLE TO WEATHER THE STORM?

DO WE HAVE TO BE DIFFERENT

SEEING LIFE A DIFFERENT WAY,

WHY DO WE HAVE TO BE DIFFERENT,

BEFORE THEY HEAR WHAT WE HAVE TO SAY.

WHAT'S WRONG WITH "DIFFERENT

WHAT'S DIFFERENT ANYWAY?

I DON'T NEED TO BE ASHAMED

BECAUSE MY WALKING GETS IN THE WAY

MY LEGS AND ARMS DON'T WORK THE

SAME

THE SAME AS ME AND YOU,

BUT EVEN IF THEY DON'T WORK RIGHT

IT DOESN'T MEAN THAT YOU

CAN'T BEAR THE SIGHT

OR STOP US STANDING UP TG FIGHT.

WE'RE JUST THE SAME AS YOU AND ME,

NO DIFFERENT, BUT YOU JUST NEED TO

SEE

BEYOND THE DIFFERENCE IS REALITY.

BEYOND REALITTY THERE'S ME

DREAMING OF WHAT I WANT TO BE

AND WHAT I HOPE YOU'LL BE ABLE TO

SEE.

(MATRON AND PETER ARE DECORATING
THE LOUNGE WITH

STREAMERS AND BALLONS, READY FOR
THE PARTY .)

PETER: Will that be all now, matron?

MATRON:I think we've just about finished. Come

along, Diane and Martin, What do you think, isn't it

looking great? I think it looks pretty super.

DIANE: That's one to go in the notebook , Martin.

Don't forget to put it down in there, now.

MATRON: Hang on, why does that need to be put

down in your famous little book that you're so fond of,

then? We never meant to cause anyone offence, it wasn't meant to be rude in any way at all.

DIANE. It's just the patronisation bit really; you always use such a condescending tone of voice. We're not two years old, and our minds STILL work properly, even if the rest of us doesn't appear to. We're just as capable of having the same thoughts and feelings as those able-bodied people out there you know, contrary to popular opinion.

MATRON:WELL…….. I NEVER had an attitude problem towards you , young lady, but it certainly looks as if you've got one almighty big chip on your shoulder, young lady.

DIANE: Here we go again. People always end up patronising us, or putting our backs up. Martin, it's definitely time for that tribunal. Peter, can you organise it for the guys out there to join in

PETER :Sure .I'll get the mic.Let's go for it and show them that you guys can have a good time in life the same as everyone else, perhaps more so.

PETER WANTDERS INTO THE AUDIENCE, HE INITIATES AN IMPROMPTUDEBATE ON STIGMA AND DISABILITY.

DRUMMING GROUP BEGIN DRUMMING, INTEGRATED WHEELCHAIR DANCING ONSTAGE.PETER INVITES MEMBERS OF THE AUDIENCE UP ONSTAGE TO JOIN IN THE DANCING.

AUDIENCE TAUGHT HOW TO SIGN TO THE TAP DANCE SONG.

FINALE   CAN CAN, WHEELCHAIR DANCERS, ABLE BODIED DANCERS AND

AUDIENCE MEMBERS DANCING ON STAGE TO

THE DRUMMING.

BALLONS LET DOWN ON STAGE, AND

ONTO THE AUDIENCE IN THE AUDITORIUM.

FIONA WHELPTON

JULY 2005.

www.ingramcontent.com/pod-product-compliance
Lightning Source LLC
Chambersburg PA
CBHW022154080426
42734CB00006B/427